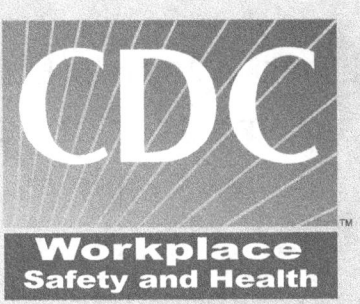

Lung Function (Spirometry) Testing in Employees at a Flavorings Manufacturing Plant --- Indiana

Kathleen Kreiss, MD
Chris Piacitelli, CIH
Jean Cox-Ganser, PhD

Health Hazard Evaluation Report
HETA 2008-0155-3131
June 2011

DEPARTMENT OF HEALTH AND HUMAN SERVICES
Centers for Disease Control and Prevention

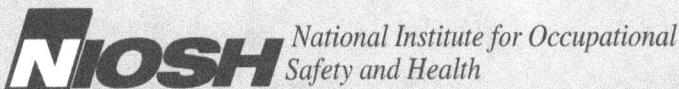 National Institute for Occupational Safety and Health

The employer shall post a copy of this report for a period of 30 calendar days at or near the workplace(s) of affected employees. The employer shall take steps to insure that the posted determinations are not altered, defaced, or covered by other material during such period. [37 FR 23640, November 7, 1972, as amended at 45 FR 2653, January 14, 1980].

CONTENTS

ABBREVIATIONS

ACOEM	American College of Occupational and Environmental Medicine
HHE	Health hazard evaluation
FEMA	Flavor and Extract Manufacturers Association
FEV_1	Forced expiratory volume in one second
FVC	Forced vital capacity
IH	Industrial hygiene
LEV	Local exhaust ventilation
LLD	Limit of longitudinal decline
LLN	Lower limit of normal
MDC	Minimum detectable concentration
mL	Milliliters
mL/year	Milliliters per year
MSDS	Material safety data sheet
NIOSH	National Institute for Occupational Safety and Health
NTIS	National Technical Information Service
OSH	Occupational Safety and Health
OSHA	Occupational Safety and Health Administration
ppm	Parts per million
RDHETAP	Respiratory Disease Hazard Evaluation and Technical Assistance Program

Introduction

The National Institute for Occupational Safety and Health (NIOSH) received a union request for a health hazard evaluation (HHE) at a flavorings manufacturing facility in Indiana. A local branch of the International Brotherhood of Teamsters submitted the HHE request because it was concerned about possible respiratory problems and the use of flavoring chemicals, including diacetyl, at the facility. NIOSH investigators conducted a site visit in May 2008 and received records of spirometry, a type of lung function test, in June 2008. After a delay incurred by litigation, the company provided additional spirometry records through September 2009, job history information for current employees, air sampling results through August 2009, and respiratory protection and hazard communications programs information.

What NIOSH Did

- NIOSH investigators visited the facility on May 29-30, 2008.

- We performed limited air sampling for volatile organic compounds at the facility and reviewed company air sampling records.

- We analyzed employees' spirometry reports in relation to work history information and assessed whether abnormalities in tests were related to work factors.

What NIOSH Found

- There were 34/106 employees (32%) with abnormal spirometry: 30/106 (28%) had a restrictive pattern of abnormality, 3/106 had an obstructive pattern and 1/106 had a mixed obstructive and restrictive pattern.

- The prevalence of restriction in most recent spirometry reports was 3.8 times higher than expected in the U.S. population.

- For the 18 employees with spirometry tests performed for all four years from 2006 to 2009, there were parallel declines in mean percent predicted forced expiratory volume in 1 second (FEV_1) and forced vital capacity (FVC) with relatively stable mean FEV_1/FVC ratio, consistent with an evolving restrictive process during employment.

- Depending on the values used to determine the threshold for abnormal decline in FEV_1 over time, between 17%-19%

of 70 employees with good quality longitudinal spirometry testing had abnormal declines.

- Five of 13 employees with excessive decline still had normal values for FEV_1, which means they would not be identified as abnormal if their repeat measurements over time were not compared to each other.

- Employees who worked in liquid compounding, process flavors, dry blend, extract and distillation, and spray dry (areas we categorized as having higher potential for flavoring exposures) had 2.8 times greater average annual declines in FEV_1 and were about 7 times more likely to have abnormal declines in FEV_1 than employees in other areas.

- The work-related declines in lung function in plant employees might be related to exposures other than diacetyl.

- Diacetyl has been measured in the air in many areas of the plant.

What Managers Can Do

- Explain to employees that there appears to be a lung hazard in this facility related to exposure to flavoring chemicals and train them to minimize exposure.

- Lower exposures to flavoring chemicals by engineering controls, work practice modifications, administrative measures, and respiratory protection until medical monitoring documents that employees are no longer at excess risk of developing occupational respiratory disease.

- Obtain baseline breathing tests (spirometry) before new employees are exposed to flavoring chemicals.

- Perform breathing tests every 3 months on all employees in areas with higher potential for exposure to flavoring chemicals and all employees with abnormal declines until abnormal declines in the work force have been controlled by lowering exposures.

- Perform breathing tests every 6 months on employees in areas with lower potential for flavoring exposures.

- Ask the occupational health clinic to refer all employees with abnormal restrictive patterns on spirometry to lung specialists for definitive tests to establish whether lung disease is the cause of restriction. All employees with abnormal obstructive patterns need referral for diagnosis, as well.

- Ask the occupational health clinic to notify employees of abnormal falls in breathing tests, even if the results remain within the normal ranges of FEV_1 and FVC. Measures should be taken as listed above to protect these employees from potentially harmful exposures. They should have follow up spirometry testing at 3 month intervals at least until their lung function has stabilized.

- Ask the occupational health clinic to analyze the spirometry findings for the whole employee population to determine whether processes continue to be associated with increased risk of abnormalities so that enhanced medical monitoring, work limitation, and exposure reduction can be implemented and prioritized.

What Employees Can Do

- Minimize exposure to flavoring chemicals.

- Use your respirator at all times when handling flavoring chemicals or near co-workers handling flavoring chemicals.

- Participate in company-scheduled breathing tests (spirometry). Ask if your lung function is declining excessively and if you have abnormalities on spirometry.

- Seek further medical evaluation if your lung function is declining excessively or if you have abnormalities on spirometry.

- Take this report to your doctor if you develop persistent cough, trouble breathing, abnormal spirometry, or abnormal drop in spirometry measurements on your latest breathing test compared to previous tests.

- Call NIOSH at 1-800-232-2114 if you have any questions about this report or your spirometry results.

Production employees at this flavoring manufacturing company had striking excesses of abnormal restrictive lung function and abnormal declines in lung function during employment. Employees with higher potential for exposure to flavorings had greater average annual decline in lung function and a 7-fold higher chance of abnormal lung function decline than employees in other areas with lower potential for exposure. Additional medical testing will be needed to determine the underlying cause(s) of these abnormalities in lung function (spirometry) testing. It is especially important to determine if those with restrictive spirometry have occupational lung disease. In the meantime, efforts should be continued to minimize exposure to diacetyl and other potentially causative inhaled agents. Those with high potential exposures should be offered ongoing medical surveillance that follows spirometry over time to assist in identifying problems that can be corrected.

In March 2008, an International Brotherhood of Teamsters local union requested a health hazard evaluation at a flavoring manufacturing company because of concern about possible lung effects of flavoring exposures, including diacetyl. In May 2008, NIOSH conducted a brief walk-through visit of the company. Subsequently, the company brought litigation to prevent further on-site evaluations. In June 2009, after resolution of the litigation, the company agreed to provide NIOSH with various medical and workplace information. All information was received by November 2009.

NIOSH staff evaluated spirometry data supplied by the company on production employees tested from 1998 through 2009. The majority of the spirometry tests was performed in the years 2004 and later. We classified spirometry tests for quality and compared the prevalence of abnormalities in acceptable quality tests to national population prevalence, adjusted for the distributions of age, sex, race, smoking, and body mass index in the company's employees. We calculated declines over time in forced expiratory volume in 1 second (FEV_1), a lung function measurement made using spirometry, for employees with more than one spirometry test of acceptable quality, since excessive decline in FEV_1 can be an early marker of lung disease. Using an approach that adjusts for quality of a spirometry monitoring program, reflected by within-person variation, we compared the declines in lung function to a statistically-determined lower limit of normal decline.

After establishing which employees had abnormal declines in lung function, we evaluated work area risk factors for associations with excessive declines in lung function, adjusted for age, smoking, tenure, change in weight, and obesity. Based on our experience in other flavoring plants, we designated a group of areas with higher potential for flavorings exposure as a possible risk factor. These were liquid compounding, process flavors, dry blend, extract and distillation, and spray dry. We compared spirometric findings for employees in these areas with employees who worked in other areas of the plant. We also evaluated environmental monitoring measurements supplied by the company before and after our walk through visit, along with the four measurements conducted during the walk through.

The flavorings manufacturing company supplied spirometry data on 112 employees; 75% of these employees had more than one test session, with a follow-up range of 0.5 to 11 years. The most recent spirometry measurement for 106 employees with at least one spirometry test of acceptable quality showed that 30/106 (28%)

employees had restrictive abnormalities, 3/106 had obstructive abnormalities, and 1/106 had both restrictive and obstructive abnormalities. The 28% of employees with restrictive abnormalities was 3.8 (95% confidence interval 2.6–5.4) times higher than would be expected in a U.S. population with the same demographic characteristics. Among the 30 employees with restrictive abnormalities, 27% had longitudinal testing demonstrating abnormal declines in FEV_1 over time, indicating that progressive deterioration in lung function had occurred; 17% had no history of longitudinal testing, and thus no evaluation for excessive decline over time was possible. In addition to the 34/106 (32%) with abnormal restrictive or obstructive spirometry, 5 employees with normal most-recent spirometry values had longitudinal testing demonstrating abnormal declines in FEV_1 over time, which, if continued, might result in spirometric abnormality. Thus a total of 39/106 (37%) employees among those with company spirometry measurements had evidence of some abnormality, either in classification of most recent spirometry as showing restriction or obstruction; and/or longitudinal spirometry showing excessive decline over time, with most recent spirometry values still within the normal range. Forty-two employees did not have serial data of adequate quality to allow evaluation for abnormal declines.

The company's 2009 exposure measurements documented that diacetyl was present in at least one sample in all sampled production areas, the laboratory, and the warehouse. Two of the four NIOSH area measurements detected diacetyl in liquid compounding and packaging areas. These findings supported our designation of a group of areas with higher potential for flavorings exposures, although some areas that were classified as being in the lower potential for exposure group did have exposures of concern.

Employees who ever worked in areas with higher potential for flavorings exposure (liquid compounding, process flavors, dry blend, extract and distillation, and spray dry) had 2.8 times greater average annual declines in FEV_1 than employees in areas with lower potential for flavorings exposure. In particular, employees who had ever worked in liquid compounding had statistically higher average annual declines in FEV_1, compared to the lower potential for exposure group. Employees who currently worked in higher potential for flavorings exposure areas were 7 times more likely to have abnormal declines in FEV_1 than employees in other areas, which is consistent with work-related risk for adverse respiratory health outcomes.

Additional medical testing is needed to determine whether the abnormal spirometry findings found among workers are due to lung disease. In particular, medical testing is needed to determine the underlying cause of restrictive spirometry. Although obesity is a major cause of restrictive abnormalities in the United States, our comparisons with the U.S. population were adjusted for the proportions of employees who were overweight or obese, as were our analyses of work area risk factors. Thus, restrictive spirometry in this workforce cannot be explained by obesity. Since the excess of spirometric abnormalities is substantial and the distribution of excessive declines in lung function is associated with history of working in areas with higher potential for exposure, there is great cause for concern about occupational lung disease. It is possible that some exposure other than diacetyl may underlie these abnormalities, since the predominant pattern of restrictive abnormalities differs from the pattern of obstructive abnormalities seen among microwave popcorn employees. Also, the flavorings used in this plant are more diverse than are found in microwave popcorn production. However, some diacetyl-exposed individuals in microwave popcorn plants and other settings have had restrictive abnormalities without other apparent cause. Thus, the spectrum of abnormalities caused by diacetyl might include restrictive lung disease. This possibility remains to be fully explored.

We recommend further lowering of flavoring exposures, without regard to anticipated exposure limits to diacetyl, since other chemicals may be associated with the adverse respiratory health outcomes documented in the workforce. We reiterate our interim report recommendations for engineering controls, work practices, enhanced respiratory protection, and medical surveillance. Ongoing medical surveillance that uses longitudinal spirometry testing to monitor those with potentially harmful exposures is also recommended, particularly until the cause of the high burden of abnormal spirometry in the workforce is fully understood. The company's contract with its medical provider should provide for aggregate epidemiologic analysis of the medical results, including analysis of medical results by department or job. Aggregate analysis can identify hazards associated with flavoring manufacture and may assist the company in targeting priorities for prevention through exposure control.

Keywords: NAICS 311930 (Flavoring Syrup and Concentrate Manufacturing), Flavorings, Diacetyl, Butter, Respiratory Symptoms, Spirometry, Restriction.

INTRODUCTION

NIOSH received an HHE request on March 19, 2008 from a local branch of the International Brotherhood of Teamsters to evaluate both the respiratory health and exposures of production employees who handle flavoring chemicals at a flavorings manufacturing facility in Indiana. While no health effects were reported, employees were concerned about exposure to flavorings including diacetyl, a butter flavoring constituent used in the facility.

BACKGROUND

Increasing cumulative exposure of workers to diacetyl has been associated with an increased prevalence of abnormal lung function [Kreiss et al. 2002; Kullman et al. 2005; NIOSH 2004]. In animal experiments conducted by NIOSH, rats exposed to vapors from diacetyl developed severe injury to their airways [Hubbs et al. 2004]. After investigating several microwave popcorn plants and finding that employees with occupational exposures to flavorings were at risk for fixed obstructive airways diseases, NIOSH disseminated an ALERT to raise awareness of the inhalation risk posed by flavorings chemicals and to provide preventive recommendations [NIOSH 2004]. Because of sufficient evidence from epidemiologic studies and animal experiments that diacetyl causes airways obstruction and excessive decline in FEV_1 [Kreiss 2007b], efforts to regulate diacetyl exposures are underway. However, the full spectrum of lung disease associated with flavoring exposures is still under investigation. In addition to obstructive lung disease, this spectrum may also include restrictive lung disease [Day et al. 2011, Akpinar-Elci et al. 2004, Kreiss 2007a].

In May 2008, NIOSH conducted an initial site visit at the facility in Indiana and at their contracted occupational clinic. The facility produces a variety of flavor formulations in liquid, paste, and powder form. Some examples of flavorings produced include butter, buttermilk, cheese, sour cream, coffee, orange, blueberry, raspberry, grape, beef, chicken, and fish. At the time of the site visit, the facility employed about 115 production employees and about 100 office employees. The production is a batch process and takes place over three shifts, five days a week. Major production areas include extract and distillation, X-Oil, liquid compounding, process flavors, dry blend, spray dry, and packaging. Other work areas include shipping, warehouse, maintenance, quality control, research and development, and administration. Arrangements were made with the occupational clinic to obtain the results of employees' spirometry, a lung function test that measures the volume and flow rate of air that can be blown out of the lungs after a full inspiration. In June 2008, we received copies of spirometry reports on facility production employees from the clinic.

Our request for an additional site visit to assess exposures, interview employees, and conduct medical tests on employees was the subject of litigation brought by the company in Federal District Court, which was concluded in May 2009. In June 2009, we issued an interim report recommending further medical and environmental evaluation. After discussions in follow up, the company agreed to provide additional medical and environmental information to NIOSH. The company provided a table of their action items in response to the interim report in August 2009, updated medical information in September and October 2009, and air sampling results in November 2009.

This final report provides results of analyses of all the spirometry records sent to NIOSH, information from the May 2008 site visit, updated information from the company, descriptions of the company's responses to the recommendations given in the interim report, and additional recommendations based on our subsequent findings.

ASSESSMENT

On May 29 and 30, 2008, NIOSH conducted an initial site visit at the facility in Indiana. The NIOSH field team for the site visit consisted of two physicians, an industrial hygienist, and a mechanical engineer. We met with union representatives, production employees, management, and attorneys. We conducted limited sampling for volatile organic compounds. On the afternoon of May 30, 2008, we visited the contracted occupational health clinic that conducts the facility's spirometry testing, medical clearance for respirator use, and respirator fit testing for its employees. While on site, we briefly reviewed available spirometry reports for 85 current employees and 4 former employees. On June 18, 2008, we received copies of the spirometry test results for 84 current and 4 former employees, allowing more detailed review. In September 2009, the flavorings company provided additional spirometry reports for 96 current employees. In addition, the company provided work history information requested by NIOSH in order to evaluate the spirometry results in relation to job. In October 2009, we requested diagnostic medical test results from the contracted clinic for any employees that had been referred for medical follow-up assessments. Some employees had been seen by a contract clinic physician to discuss abnormal spirometry results, but we received no additional information about diagnostic testing done to determine the cause of abnormal spirometry results. In November 2009, the company provided updated air sampling results and information on their respiratory protection and hazard communication programs.

Demographic information

We abstracted information from spirometry records on gender and race, as well as the age, height, and weight of each employee on their test date. The spirometry records usually provided information on smoking status at the time of the test (Y/N). We used this smoking status data to create a dichotomous smoking variable, which indicated whether or not a person was ever categorized as a smoker at any testing interval.

Work history information

In September 2009, we received work history information for 97 current and former employees. Work history information included job title and the start dates for each job title. The work history also indicated if a person had been terminated. We had spirometry records but no work history information for 15 employees. We had work history information but no spirometry record for 1 employee.

We used the dates in the work history information to calculate total tenure in years. The job titles supplied by the company identified the area where the employee worked and the job he/she performed in that area. There were 12 areas identified: administration, dry blend, extract and distillation, liquid compounding, maintenance, packaging, process flavors, sample ordering, spray dry, warehouse, quality control, and research and development. Because a relatively small number of people worked in the quality control and research and development areas and because it is likely that employees in these two areas experienced similar levels of exposure to flavoring chemicals, we combined the quality control and research and development areas into one category for our analyses. Based on information obtained from the site visit about where liquid and dry flavorings were produced and on work history information provided by the company, we assigned employees in the following areas to the category of higher potential for exposure to flavoring chemicals: dry blend, extract and distillation, liquid compounding, process flavors, and spray dry.

We categorized the work history information four different ways: (1) currently working in an area; (2) ever worked in an area; (3) currently working in areas with higher vs. lower potential for exposure; (4) ever worked in areas with higher vs. lower potential for exposure. During the site visit in May 2008, the company provided a list of employees scheduled to work that day and a list of employees' last spirometry results, which included information about which area the employees worked in. This information was used to supplement missing data for the 15 employees without work history information so they could be included in our 'ever worked in an area' analyses.

Spirometry records evaluation

We evaluated 369 spirometry records measuring exhaled air volumes and flow rates achieved during a maximal forced expiration after a full inspiration from a total of 112 employees. The records dated from July 6, 1998 to August 25, 2009. Information from the records was entered into a database using a double entry system for quality control. We used SAS® (version 9.2, SAS Institute Inc., Cary, North Carolina, United States) statistical software to analyze the data.

Two-thirds of the spirometry tests were performed using an EasyOne™ spirometer (ndd Medical Technologies, Andover, Massachusetts). The test reports for most of these included a quality grade. When reports did not include a quality grade (as was the case for 29 tests performed using an EasyOne spirometer and for 119 tests performed with another type of spirometer), we graded spirometry using the EasyOne Spirometry EasyGuide criteria from the version 4.0 manual. Spirometry tests graded A and B had at least three acceptable expiratory efforts, and measurements for FEV_1 and FVC matched within 200 milliliters (mL) or less. Spirometry tests graded C had at least two acceptable efforts, and measurements for FEV_1 and FVC matched within 250 mL or less. Spirometry tests graded D had only one acceptable effort, or the two best acceptable measurements did not meet the 250 mL criterion for repeatability. Spirometry graded F had no acceptable efforts. There were four tests performed with a different model spirometer that did not have enough information about each individual expiratory effort to allow for a quality grade to be assigned.

To classify whether employees' spirometry test results were normal or abnormal, we compared each employee's most recent spirometry test results to reference values (based on age, height, gender, and race) using a reference equation developed from U.S. population data from the Third National Health and Nutrition Examination Survey [Hankinson et al. 1999].[1] For some individuals with more than one spirometry report, substantial variation was noted in recorded heights. For these individuals, we used the most frequently recorded height value (mode) to interpret spirometry results. When there was no mode height value, we used the mean of the reported heights.

Spirometry results with A, B, or C quality grade were able to be interpreted as normal or abnormal. If a test had a D quality grade but documented normal ventilatory function, it was interpreted as normal. If a test of D quality was consistent with abnormal ventilatory function, it was considered uninterpretable, because it was not possible to say if this finding was real or an artifact of poor test quality. If a test had an F quality grade, the test was considered uninterpretable. We classified abnormalities in spirometry test results as obstructive, restrictive, or mixed obstructive and restrictive (described below). We further categorized such abnormalities as mild, moderate, moderately severe, severe, or very severe based on the most recent guidance on interpreting lung function tests [Pellegrino et al. 2005].

In an obstructive pattern of abnormal spirometry, air is exhaled from the lungs more slowly than normal, as can be found in asthma, bronchitis, emphysema, and bronchiolitis obliterans. It is defined by an FEV_1 below the lower limit of normal (LLN) and a reduced ratio of FEV_1 to the total volume of air blown out of the chest during the forced expiration (FEV_1/FVC). The greater the obstruction, the more difficult it is to exhale the air from the lungs. Individuals with evidence of airways obstruction on spirometry testing can be given a bronchodilator medication, followed by repeat spirometry, to see if the obstruction is reversible,

1   The National Health and Nutrition Examination Survey is a program of studies designed to assess the health and nutritional status of adults and children in the United States. The survey combines interviews and physical examinations. It is a major program of the National Center for Health Statistics, a part of the Centers for Disease Control and Prevention. Information can be found at: http://www.cdc.gov/nchs/nhanes.htm

as is characteristic of asthma. In contrast, the obstruction found in flavoring-exposed individuals with bronchiolitis obliterans is irreversible.

In a restrictive pattern of abnormal spirometry, the total amount of air exhaled is smaller than normal. Thus, this abnormality is defined by an FVC below the LLN, with a normal FEV_1/FVC ratio. This type of abnormal spirometry often reflects a decreased volume of air in the lungs at full inspiration. It can occur in people with stiff lungs, such as is found in pulmonary fibrosis (lung scarring); people with weak respiratory muscles; or people who are considerably overweight. The greater the restriction, the greater will be the possible physical limitation.

A mixed obstructive/restrictive pattern of abnormal spirometry is defined by an FVC below the LLN, with an FEV_1/FVC ratio that is also below the LLN. A mixed pattern of abnormal spirometry can be seen in people who have severe airways disease in the absence of lung scarring, respiratory muscle weakness, or obesity; and in people with more than one type of disease process affecting the lungs.

We compared the prevalence of an abnormal restrictive pattern of spirometry with the prevalence that would be expected in the U.S. general population with the same distributions of age (less than 40 years and 40 or older), sex, race, ethnicity, ever smoking (yes, no) and body mass index (less than 25, 25 to less than 30, and 30 or greater kilograms/meters^2), which is a classification of overweight and obesity. The U.S. population prevalences were based on the third National Health and Nutrition Examination Survey [National Center for Health Statistics 1996].

Changes in lung function over time

In adulthood, it is normal for lung function to decline slowly as a person ages. After achieving highest levels of FEV_1, sometimes as late as in their thirties, individuals lose about 20-30 mL/year on average [Sherrill et al. 1992]. An excessive rate of FEV_1 decline can indicate developing lung disease. The ability to reliably detect small increases in rate of FEV_1 decline, especially over time intervals of less than about 7 years, is influenced by the quality of spirometry. If the quality of spirometry is low, measurements of FEV_1 are less precise, and it may not be possible to determine if small changes are real or artifactual. For employees having spirometry on more than one occasion, we investigated changes in lung function over time using spirometry tests of A, B, or C quality.

As a first approach to investigating lung function changes over time, we estimated population average changes in FEV_1 and FVC as mL/year. Individual values used to calculate these averages were determined by linear regression of all the FEV_1 and FVC values against time for each employee who had spirometry results available for more than one point in time.

As a second approach, we identified individuals with excessive changes in FEV_1 over time using software developed by NIOSH for longitudinal spirometry analysis (SPIROLA) [Hnizdo et al. 2010]. For individuals with less than 8 years of follow-up, this program compares FEV_1 values to the limit of longitudinal decline (LLD). The LLD is a threshold value used to determine whether the lung function decline between the first FEV_1 value (or a mean of the first two observations, if the first FEV_1 value is lower than the second one) and each follow-up FEV_1 value is excessive. Observations that fall below the LLD warrant concern as having less than a 5% chance of being normal. Beginning with 8 years of follow-up, SPIROLA bases the interpretation of excessive decline on an individual's regression slope and the lower 95% confidence limit around the regression line.

The SPIROLA software adjusts its determination of LLD for spirometry quality, as reflected by within-person variation, in addition to considering what would be normal declines in healthy persons. Unusually high quality spirometry monitoring programs, often carried out for research purposes, can achieve a within-person variation of approximately 3% [Wang and Petsonk, 2004; Wang et al. 2006]. We determined that the employees' spirometry data of A, B, and C quality had a within-person variability of 5%. We used SPIROLA to identify an LLD of 12.4% longitudinal decline based on the relative within-person variation of 5% and a referential rate of FEV_1 decline of 30 mL/year.

At the suggestion of the company in an August 2009 letter, we repeated the SPIROLA analysis using the American College of Occupational and Environmental Medicine (ACOEM) limit of longitudinal decline calculated as LLD = (Baseline $FEV_1 \times 0.85$) - (# of years × 30 mL/year), based on 15% longitudinal decline and a referential rate of decline of 30 mL/year. This limit requires an individual to have greater rate of decline in FEV_1 in order to be classified as abnormal. Thus, it is more specific but less sensitive for detecting abnormal decline. This more stringent LLD is appropriate in settings where spirometry is of relatively poor quality. However, because it is not statistically-based, it does not adjust the LLD threshold for better quality programs and their ability to measure FEV_1 with greater precision.

Associations between work history and lung function

An uneven distribution of abnormal medical test results within a working population suggests that some areas or jobs may have higher risk. We investigated possible associations between lung function and the work area variables in two ways. Using logistic regression, we modeled the presence of restrictive abnormalities based on the most recent spirometry test and having excessive FEV_1 decline as categorical variables against work area. Secondly, we used analysis of variance models to investigate the association of changes in FEV_1 and FVC as continuous variables with work area variables. Both types of models were adjusted for body mass index of 30 or more kilogram/meters^2 (obesity or not) at the last test, change in weight over the spirometry testing period for each employee (as pounds per year), age at last test, smoking as a yes or no categorical variable, and tenure in years. For the models using ever worked in any one specific area with higher potential for flavoring exposure, we used those who never worked in the areas with higher potential for exposure to flavoring chemicals as the comparison group. Similarly, we compared current employees in any one specific area with higher potential for exposure to the employees not currently working in areas with higher potential for exposure.

Exposure assessment

The company completed a form about the frequency of use and annual poundage for the 34 flavoring substances on the Flavor and Extract Manufacturers Association (FEMA) high priority list [FEMA 2004], starter distillate, limonene, nonane, and any other chemicals used in large quantities. FEMA had classified 83 flavoring substances as priorities for consideration as potentially posing respiratory hazards in flavoring manufacturing workplaces. The priority levels were assigned based on inhalation exposure data in animals and humans, chemical structure, and volatility. FEMA stated that the 34 substances classified as high priority chemicals may pose a risk of respiratory injury when associated with high exposure levels, repeated low exposure levels, heating, or inadequate controls. The form also collected information on the form (solid, liquid, or paste) of each chemical used and examples of product flavors in which the chemical was used.

We reviewed company reports of air sampling conducted by their industrial hygiene consultants between March 2004 and July 2007 and between July 2008 and August 2009.

During our site visit, we collected 4 air samples for volatile organic compound screening, each for about an hour, in the liquid compounding, spray dry and dry blend, quality control laboratory, and packaging areas. The samples were collected on stainless steel thermal desorption tubes containing 3 beds of sorbent material at a flow rate of 50 milliliters per minute and analyzed per NIOSH Method 2549 [NIOSH 2008] using thermal desorption, gas chromatography, and mass spectrometry. These samples do not give quantitative measurements, but do provide qualitative results which indicate relative abundance of a wide range of compounds found in the air. NIOSH investigators typically use this approach to collect information to help guide a more in-depth exposure assessment.

Engineering controls

We observed engineering controls (e.g., local exhaust ventilation hoods) in several areas throughout the facility during our site visit.

Respiratory protection

Prior to our May 2008 site visit, we received a copy of the company's respiratory protection program documentation. During our visit, we interviewed production employees, managers, and supervisors about their knowledge and use of respirators, and we reviewed 2004-2008 respirator fit-testing records at the contracted occupational health clinic. The company sent us a copy of their August 2009 respiratory protection program in November 2009.

Hazard communication

During the site visit, we reviewed the written hazard communication program and material safety data sheets (MSDSs) for two of the company's diacetyl-containing products. In November 2009, we received a copy of the company's July 2009 hazard communication program.

Demographic information

The demographic information for the employees is given in Table 1.

Table 1. Demographic characteristics for 112 flavorings manufacturing facility employees

Gender (male), n (%)	96 (85.7)
Race, n (%)	
Caucasian	86 (76.8)
Black	23 (20.5)
Hispanic	3 (2.7)
Ever smoked (yes),* n (%)	32 (29.6)
Age in years‡, mean (range)	45.5 (21–67)
Tenure† in years‡, mean (range)	16.2 (0.64–36.1)
Body Mass Index > = 30 kg/m^2, n‡ (%)	33 (29.5)

*Smoking status was available for 108 employees.
‡Calculated on date of most recent spirometry test date; for tenure the calculation is years from hire date to most recent spirometry test date
†Tenure information available for 95 employees

Work history information

Table 2 shows the number of employees who currently and ever worked in each of the areas identified in the company-provided information. Extract and distillation was only mentioned as a work area for one employee in the past and for none currently. It may be that the terminology for that department or area has changed over time. There were six employees who had formerly been in administration.

Table 2. Work area distribution of employees with spirometry and work history data

Work area	Number of employees currently	Number of employees ever
Administration	0	6
Dry blend*	7	20
Extract and distillation*	0	1
Liquid compounding*	22	47
Maintenance	7	16
Packaging	19	49
Process flavors*	9	16
QC and R&D†	12	20
Sample order	3	3
Spray dry*	4	8
Warehouse	14	27
Total	97	

*In our analyses, an area defined as having higher potential for flavoring exposure in comparison to other work areas.
†Quality Control and Research Development

Evaluation of spirometry records

After we combined all spirometry records provided to NIOSH, there were spirometry reports for 112 employees. Table 3 shows the number of reports by year of testing and according to spirometry test quality. The number of available test results is much greater starting in 2004 than earlier. Figure 1 shows the distribution of spirometry follow-up time for the 112 employees. This ranged from 0 months to 11 years. Twenty-eight employees had one spirometry test available, and 84 employees had more than one spirometry test available. Seventy employees had two or more spirometry tests of A, B, or C quality, and 66 of these also had work area information. The group of 45 employees with at least two spirometry reports who had ever worked in areas of higher potential for flavoring exposures had an average follow-up of 5.4 years, in comparison to 3.5 years follow-up for the group of 21 employees in areas with lower exposure potential. The 28 employees who were currently working in areas of higher potential for flavoring exposure had an

Table 3. Number and quality of spirometry test reports for flavorings manufacturing facility employees by year of testing

Year	A-C quality	D quality	F quality/no quality reported or able to be created
1998	4	1	3
1999	7	1	0
2000	0	0	0
2001	1	0	0
2002	0	0	0
2003	0	0	0
2004	27	3	0
2005	20	9	0
2006	41	5	0
2007	50	9	1
2008	75	12	4
2009	77	18	1
Totals	302	58	9

Figure 1. Distribution of 112 flavoring manufacturing employees by years of spirometry follow-up.

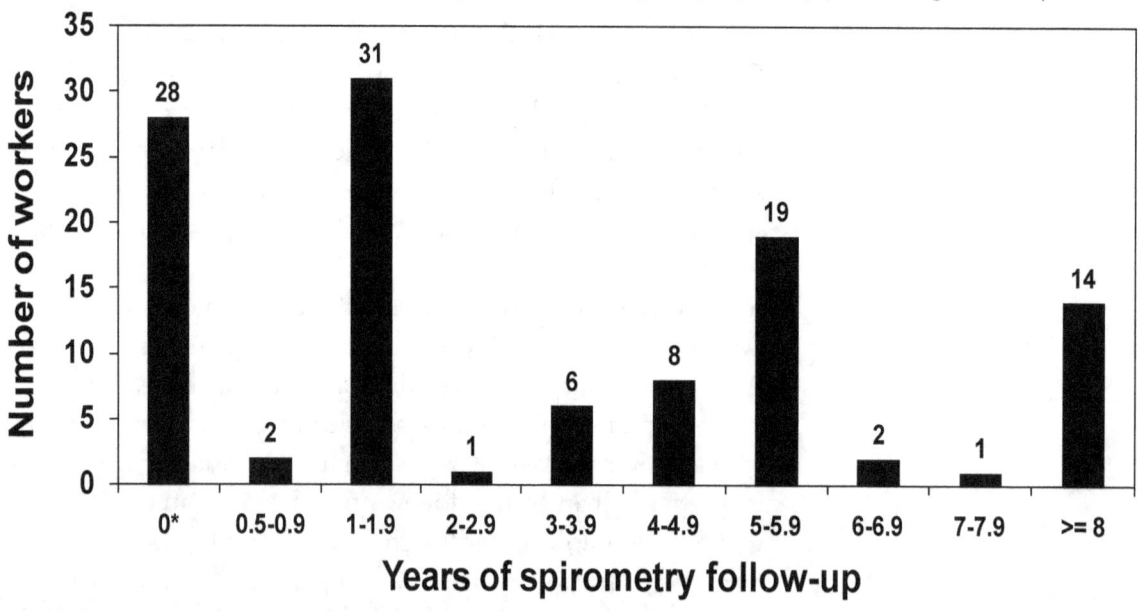

* This indicates having only 1 spirometry test.

average of 5.6 years of follow-up, compared to 4.4 years of follow-up for the 35 employees with lower current potential for exposure.

Interpretation of most recent spirometry tests

The most recent test was performed in 2009 for 96 employees, in 2008 for 12 employees and between 2004 and 2006 for four employees. Forty-eight percent of the most recent spirometry tests for each individual had A quality, 14% had B quality, 18% had C quality, 18% had D quality, and 2% had F quality. We interpreted 106 of the 112 tests (90 of A-C quality and 16 of D quality with a normal interpretation). We identified 34/106 (32%) employees as having abnormal spirometry results. We found a restrictive pattern in 30/106 (28%) employees (22 mild abnormality, six moderate abnormality, one moderately severe abnormality, and one severe abnormality). Additionally, we identified two employees with mild obstruction, one employee with moderate obstruction, and one with a very severe mixed pattern on their most recent spirometry test (Table 4).

Table 4. NIOSH interpretation of most recent spirometry tests from employees at a flavorings manufacturing facility

Interpretation	Employees N = 106* n (%)
Normal	72 (68%)
Restricted	30 (28%)
Mild	22 (21%)
Moderate	6 (6%)
Moderately severe	1 (1%)
Severe	1 (1%)
Obstructed	3 (3%)
Mild	2 (2%)
Moderate	1 (1%)
Mixed	1 (1%)
Very severe	1 (1%)

*Tests were considered interpretable as normal or abnormal if the quality was A, B, or C. Additionally, D quality tests achieving values in the normal range were interpreted as normal. D quality tests with values in the abnormal range were considered uninterpretable because of the possibility that abnormal values were due to poor test quality. If a test had an F quality, the test was considered uninterpretable. There were 6 such tests.

The number of restrictive spirometry abnormalities seen in these employees is high. Company employees with spirometry measurements had 3.8 times the prevalence of abnormal restriction compared to the U.S. population adjusted for age, gender, race, ever smoking, and body mass index (prevalence ratio 3.8; 95% confidence limit 2.6-5.4). For this analysis, we excluded four employees for whom we did not have smoking information.

Changes in lung function over time

Average longitudinal decline of FEV_1 and FVC were similar in magnitude and larger than would be expected due to aging. As calculated using the slopes of the regression of lung function over time for A, B, or C quality tests, the mean decline in FEV_1 was 77 mL/year and the mean decline in FVC was 89 mL/year for non-smokers (n = 46). For ever smokers (n = 22), these values were 109 mL/year for FEV_1 and 147 mL/year for FVC. Results for percent predicted FEV_1 and FVC (which adjust for age) for the 18 employees tested for all four years from 2006 to 2009 showed parallel declines in average percent predicted FEV_1 and FVC over time with relatively stable FEV_1/FVC ratio (Figure 2), consistent with a tendency toward restriction.

Figure 2. Group means of percent predicted FVC and FEV_1 and FEV_1/FVC ratio by year of test for all A-C quality spirometry tests for 18 employees tested 2006 - 2009. If there was more than 1 test per worker in a year, the last test of the year was used.

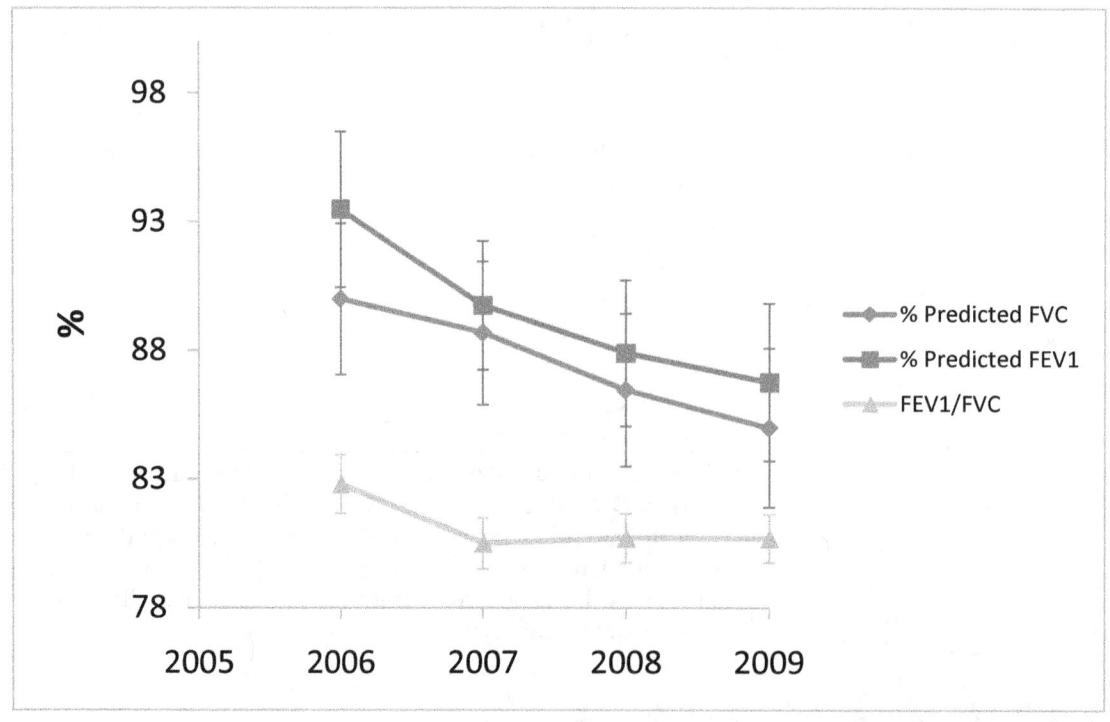

There were 70 employees with two or more spirometry tests of A, B, or C quality used in the SPIROLA analyses of abnormal declines in FEV_1 using criteria for determination of LLD that adjusted for 5% within-person variability. Of these 70 employees, 13 (19%) were identified as having excessive FEV_1 declines using the 12.4% longitudinal decline criterion. The employee with abnormal decline and the shortest period of follow-up (1.9 years) lost 499 mL/year, for a total of 900 mL in FEV_1. The others with abnormal declines in FEV_1 had abnormal declines over 4.3 to 10.7 years with annualized declines of 92-188 mL/year. Of these 13 employees who had experienced abnormal rates of decline, five continued to have FEV_1 values in the normal range at their most recent spirometry test. These employees may need interventions to prevent them from declining further into the abnormal range of lung function. We found that 8 (32%) of 25 employees with both abnormal restrictive spirometry and serial measurements had excessive decline in FEV_1, suggesting that the abnormality was progressing.

Using the more stringent value of LLD based on ACOEM recommendations, 12 of 70 employees (17%) were identified as having excessive FEV_1 declines. Five of these employees had a normal value of FEV_1 at their latest spirometry test.

In summary, 30 employees had restriction on spirometry, three had obstruction, and one had a mixed pattern, and an additional 5 employees had excessive FEV_1 declines within the normal range of spirometry, for a total of 39 employees (37%) with either abnormal spirometry, an excessive decline in FEV_1, or both. Only 63% of employees had serial spirometry of adequate quality to evaluate excessive FEV_1 declines, so these proportions of the workforce with spirometric findings suggestive of lung disease may be low. Use of the 15% ACOEM criterion for excessive decline did not substantially change how many individuals were identified as having excessive decline in FEV_1 compared to use of a statistically determined threshold.

Associations between work history and lung function

Since employees in the facility had more abnormalities than we expected, both in spirometric restriction and in abnormal rapid decline in FEV_1, we examined possible work-relatedness by examining if employees with higher potential for exposure to flavorings were more affected.

Restriction on last spirometry showed no significant associations with work area. Changes in FEV_1 and FVC in mL/year were associated ($p < 0.05$) with ever having worked in areas with higher potential for exposure to flavorings. The adjusted means for change in FEV_1 for ever worked in higher potential exposure areas versus never having worked in these areas were -124 mL/year compared to -44 mL/year, while for changes in FVC, these values were -144 mL/year compared to -63 mL/year. Within the category of higher potential for exposure, ever having worked in liquid compounding, as compared to never having worked in areas with higher potential for exposure, was associated with a larger decline in FEV_1 (adjusted means of -118 mL/year vs. -47 mL/year; $p < 0.05$). Decline in FVC showed a trend for a larger decline for those who had ever worked in liquid compounding (adjusted means of -138 mL/year vs. -69 mL/year; $p < 0.1$).

Excessive decline in FEV_1, defined in comparison to a 12.4% longitudinal decline plus a referential decline of 30 mL/year, was associated with currently working in higher potential for exposure areas (odds ratio = 7.0; 95% confidence interval = 1.3-38.2, $p < 0.05$) and marginally associated with ever working in higher potential for exposure areas (odds ratio = 7.5; 95% confidence interval = 0.99-56.7, $p < 0.1$). Consistent results with regard to trend were found when excessive decline in FEV_1 was defined with the ACOEM 15% criteria (Table 5).

Table 5. Associations between excessive decline in FEV_1 and working in areas with higher potential for exposure to flavorings*†

Excessive decline criterion	Ever worked in area with higher potential for exposure Odds ratio (95% confidence limit)	Currently working in area with higher potential for exposure Odds ratio (95% confidence limit)
12.4% longitudinal decline and referential decline of 30 mL/year ‡	7.5 (0.99-56.7)§	7.0 (1.3-38.2) ¶
15% longitudinal decline and referential decline of 30 mL/year	8.3 (0.99-69.8)§	6.9 (1.2-40.9) ¶

*Logistic models adjusted for body mass index at time of most recent test equal to or greater than 30 or not, change in weight over the spirometry testing period for each employee (as pounds per year), age at last test, smoking as a yes or no categorical variable, and tenure in years.
†Summary includes spirometry tests with quality grade of A, B, or C.
‡This uses the estimated within person variability of 5%.
§$p < 0.1$
¶$p < 0.05$

RESULTS (CONTINUED)

Exposure assessment

The company reported using 24 of the 34 FEMA high priority substances, as well as starter distillate and limonene, and most substances were in liquid form. Nine of the 24 were used on a frequent basis (Table 6). No information was received for other chemicals (not on the FEMA list) used in large quantities.

Table 6. Flavoring substances used in production at flavorings manufacturing facility by frequency of use, June 2008*

Flavoring substance	Frequency of use† 1 = rarely, 5 = often, 10 = daily
USED FREQUENTLY	
Acetaldehyde	9
Acetic acid	9
Acetoin	9
Benzaldehyde	9
Butyric acid	9
Diacetyl	9
Furfural	7
Limonene ‡	7
Phosphoric acid	9
Propionic acid	7
Starter distillate ‡	5
USED LESS FREQUENTLY	
Ammonium sulfide	2
Ethyl acrylate	1
Formic acid	3
Hydrogen sulfide	1
Isobutyraldehyde	3
Isobutyric acid	3
Methyl mercaptan	3
2-Pentenal	1
Phenol	1
Piperidine	1
Propionaldehyde	3
Pyridine	2
Pyrrolidine	2
Trimethylamine	3
Valeraldehyde	3

* Information received for substances listed on a request form after the site visit. Field for "Other ingredients used in large quantities" was left blank.
†Request form provided the three categorical frequency ranking choices. Company responded with frequency ranking on a continuous scale between 0 and 10.
‡ All substances in table except these are on the FEMA High Priority Substance list [FEMA 2004]. Ten other substances on the list and nonane were not used.

Between March 2004 and July 2007, the facility's industrial hygiene consultants performed four air sampling evaluations at the plant when diacetyl-containing products were being prepared (Table 7). Sampled analytes included acetaldehyde, acetic acid, benzyl alcohol, butyric acid, diacetyl, ethyl acetate, ethyl alcohol, phosphoric acid, respirable dust, and total dust. For all substances that have occupational exposure guidelines, none were found at levels above the guideline limits. NIOSH Method 2557 was used to sample for diacetyl in the X-Oil room, liquid compounding, spray dry, packaging, and laboratory areas. Diacetyl was found above the limit of detection in the X-Oil room, liquid compounding, and spray dry, at 8-hour time-weighted average concentrations up to 10.2 parts per million (ppm) for area samples and 0.7 ppm for personal samples (Table 7). NIOSH Method 2557 has been found to be affected by humidity, diacetyl concentration, and time to sample extraction [Cox-Ganser et al. 2011], so these results are likely underestimates of the true values.

Table 7. Company diacetyl air sampling results using NIOSH Method 2557* from March 2004 to July 2007

Sample Type	Location	Number of samples	Number of samples less than MDC[†]	8-hour time-weighted average concentration[‡] (ppm)[§]		
				Minimum	Maximum	Geometric mean[¶]
Area	Laboratory	3	3	< 0.030**	< 0.030	< 0.015
Area	Liquid compounding	2	1	< 0.028	10.165	0.375
Area	Packaging	2	2	< 0.015	< 0.015	< 0.007
Area	Spray dry	1	0	0.169	0.169	0.169
Area	X-Oil[††]	5	1	< 0.033	3.208	0.258
Personal	Liquid compounding	4	3	< 0.029	0.260	0.030
Personal	Liquid compounding and X-Oil	1	1	< 0.029	< 0.029	< 0.015
Personal	Packaging	1	1	< 0.015	< 0.015	< 0.008
Personal	Spray dry	2	0	0.056	0.269	0.123
Personal	X-Oil[††]	1	0	0.762	0.762	0.762

*NIOSH Method 2557 is affected by humidity, diacetyl concentration, and days to sample extraction, so these concentrations may be underestimates.

[†]MDC = minimum detectable concentration

[‡]Company results converted to 8-hour time-weighted averages with assumption of no exposure during unsampled periods of the shift.

[§]ppm = parts diacetyl per million parts air

[¶]All values less than MDC were replaced with MDC/2 for calculation of geometric means.

**The symbol < indicates concentration was not detectable; value presented is the MDC for minimum–maximums and MDC/2 for geometric means.

[††]Two additional samples (0.89 ppm area, 3.00 ppm personal) were reported without sufficient data (sampling volume and time) to calculate 8-hour time-weighted averages.

In the limited NIOSH air sampling, diacetyl was found in both the liquid compounding and packaging areas (Table 8). Acetoin was only seen in liquid compounding. Ethyl acetate, ethyl butyrate, benzaldehyde, limonene, $C_{10}H_{16}$ terpenes, and trichloroethylene were identified in most areas sampled. Overall, 61 compounds were identified in the four samples.

Table 8. Results from thermal desorption tubes collected by NIOSH investigators on May 29, 2008

Location	Sampling duration (minutes)	Major peaks detected*	Surroundings/job activity
Liquid compounding	60	Diacetyl Acetoin derivatives Ethyl acetate Ethyl butyrate Benzaldehyde Limonene Propylene glycol Trichloroethylene	Sample collected approximately 5 feet from a liquid compounding station making a lemon emulsion formula in the small open area adjacent to the liquid compounding room. We did not observe other activities being performed during this sampling.
Spray dry & dry blend	55	Limonene Trichloroethylene	A dry blend operation was producing a beef savory mix with the sample collected approximately 5 feet from the mixer. The NIOSH industrial hygienist could not find the batch order to identify ingredients.
Quality control laboratory	53	Ethyl acetate Ethyl butyrate Benzaldehyde Limonene $C_{10}H_{16}$ terpenes Trichloroethylene	Two laboratory personnel were performing multiple lab tests on two separate bench tops. The sample was collected on the middle bench located in the middle of the room. We did not observe other operations being performed during this sampling.
Packaging	58	Diacetyl Ethyl acetate Ethyl butyrate Benzaldehyde Limonene $C_{10}H_{16}$ terpenes Trichloroethylene	Two production lines were packaging liquid product. We observed multiple individuals operating the lines. One line was packaging an Orange/Mango product (primary ingredients could not be located), and the other product was not identified by the NIOSH industrial hygienist.

*None of the compounds reported in this table were detected on the field blank.

Table 9 presents company results from area and personal air sampling for diacetyl from production areas, laboratories, and the warehouse on 17 days between July 2008 and August 2009. The company reported that the sampling was performed either for periodic monitoring or to evaluate effectiveness of engineering and administrative controls. The samples were collected using Occupational Safety and Health Administration (OSHA) Method PV2118 on the first 2 days of sampling and OSHA Method 1012 on the remainder of sampling days beginning in March 2009. All areas sampled had detectable levels of diacetyl, at 8-hour

Table 9. Company air sampling results using OSHA Methods PV2118 and 1012 from July 2008 to August 2009

Sample Type	Location	Number of samples	Number of samples less than MDC[†]	8-hour time-weighted average concentration[‡] (ppm)[§]		
				Minimum	Maximum	Geometric mean[¶]
Diacetyl Samples						
Area	Area 25	2	0	0.073	0.073	0.073
Area	Coffee & tea	15	5	0.015[††]	0.395	0.076
Area	Dry blend	3	0	0.001	0.799	0.008
Area	Laboratory	9	4	0.001[††]	< 0.060[**]	0.002
Area	Liquid compounding	5	1	0.007[††]	< 0.060	0.014
Area	Packaging	7	1	0.001[††]	< 0.060	0.002
Area	Spray dry	5	0	0.042	2.917	0.167
Area	Tallow	3	0	0.037	0.042	0.039
Area	Warehouse	2	0	0.001	0.002	0.001
Area	X-Oil	20	3	0.008[††]	0.421	0.055
Personal	Coffee & tea	14	6	0.018[††]	< 0.975	0.155
Personal	Coffee & tea / X-Oil	1	0	0.587	0.587	0.587
Personal	Dry blend	4	0	0.002	0.219	0.011
Personal	Laboratory	9	5	< 0.001	0.027	0.003
Personal	Liquid compounding	1	0	1.900	1.900	1.900
Personal	Packaging	5	2	0.001[††]	< 0.118	0.007
Personal	Spray dry	3	0	0.076	0.457	0.182
Personal	Tallow	1	0	0.892	0.892	0.892
Personal	X-Oil	7	1	0.001[††]	1.000	0.093
Acetoin Samples						
Area	X-Oil	2	2	< 0.0002	< 0.060‡	< 0.002
Personal	X-Oil	2	0	0.003	0.510	0.036

†MDC = minimum detectable concentration

‡Most company results provided as 8-hour time-weighted average concentrations; when not, company results converted to 8-hour time-weighted averages with assumption of no exposure during unsampled periods of the shift.

§ppm = parts diacetyl per million parts air

¶All values less than MDC were replaced with MDC/2 for calculation of geometric means.

**The symbol < indicates concentration was not detectable; value presented is the MDC for minimum–maximums and MDC/2 for geometric means.

††The value presented was a detectable concentration; other samples in the set were not detectable and had MDCs higher than this value.

time-weighted average concentrations up to 2.9 ppm for area samples and 1.9 ppm for personal samples. The areas with higher maximum diacetyl concentrations were in coffee and tea, dry blend, spray dry, X-Oil, liquid compounding, and tallow, all of which are presumably in the five areas with potentially higher risk for exposure that we used in our work-related analyses. The highest levels of diacetyl measured in air samples from the laboratory and packaging areas were concerning, even though the averages of the samples were quite low. Also included in Table 9 are acetoin air sampling results; one personal sample measured an 8-hour time-weighted average concentration of 0.51 ppm.

Engineering controls

In 2008, we observed several local exhaust ventilation (LEV) hoods during our site visit. These controls included moveable exhaust hoods (also known as elephant trunk or snorkel hoods), mixing tank ventilation, ribbon blender exhaust, and spray dryer packaging exhaust hoods.

Moveable exhaust hoods were being used in many areas throughout the plant, including liquid compounding, dry blend, and spray dry. These hoods were often located near bench-top workstations on an adjustable arm which allows the employee to position the LEV to accommodate varying procedures on the bench. We observed a few of these hoods raised to levels that would make it difficult for an employee to easily grab and position the hood near the process. These hoods provided a flexible mechanism to collect contaminants and control exposures. However, their effectiveness would have been dramatically affected by cross drafts, and capture velocity would drop off quickly as distance increased between the contaminant source and the hood face. We also observed a number of fans throughout the facility, which was not air-conditioned. The fans were reportedly used as a method to cool the employees at times of high heat and humidity. However, these fans could have disturbed the airflow and dramatically reduced the effectiveness of LEV hoods, particularly the moveable exhaust hoods. In response to our recommendations concerning LEV hood performance, design or operational deficiencies, fan use, cooling methods, and negative pressure in production areas, the company indicated in their action items that they had made changes addressing hood performance and eliminated fans in X-Oil room, spray dry, and blending (Table 10).

Table 10. Flavorings manufacturing facility action items as reproduced from August 2009 company response to the interim report

Item No.	Action Item	Proposed Action	Estimated Completion Date	Status
1	Define compliance gaps relative to proposed OSHA Diacetyl standard.	Perform gap analysis.	08-Jun-09	Complete. Action items incorporated into this list.
2	Develop personnel and area sampling plan and schedule.	Design chart to report all results. Develop schedule for sampling in the production, warehouse, QC, SOD, and R&D areas.	TBD	Sampling phase I completed. Sampling phase II started week of July 13th after improved ventilation in X-oil room, testing of a closed pumping system for pure diacetyl, and implementation of improved procedures.
3	Repeat study to define adequacy of local exhaust ventilation in rooms, where diacetyl is transferred.	Conduct test and follow-up on the findings.	17-Jun-09	Testing conducted and all systems confirmed to be operating properly. Certificates posted at all primary ventilation points.
4	Evaluate X-Oil room ventilation.	Test & certify air exchanges.	17-Jun-09	Testing conducted and all systems confirmed to be operating properly. Certificates posted at all primary ventilation points.
5	Check for negative ventilation in diacetyl use production areas.	Obtain smoke tubes and perform tests at interfaces. Determine feasibility of providing negative ventilation.	17-Jun-09	Complete. Floor fans will not be used in areas diacetyl is dispensed. Procedure implemented in X-oil room to discontinue use of fans.
6	Define effect of floor fans on ventilation efficiency.	Perform smoke test at dispensing stations with and without fans operating. Develop procedures as needed to ensure adequate ventilation performance.	17-Jun-09	Complete. Floor fans will not be used in areas where diacetyl is dispensed. Procedure implemented in X-oil room to discontinue use of fans. Use of floor/ceiling fans in Spray Dry and Blending will also be discontinued.
7	Develop closed system handling of diacetyl.	Modify diacetyl transfer equipment and procedures to minimize potential exposure during diacetyl transfers.	24-Jun-09	Pump system currently being tested to achieve a closed dispensing system. Plan to develop a complete dispensing, receiving, mixing system, if sampling results show need.
8	Define current handling procedures for diacetyl in the labs.	Labs report use, quantity, and dispensing methods.	22-Jun-09	Complete. All lab staff using ventilation systems and hoods. Procedures updated to reflect proposed OSHA standard and personnel trained on the procedure.
9	Evaluate adequacy of respirators currently used.	Contact supplier for protection factor and assess level of protection. Complete analysis when the sampling program is implemented.	16-Jun-09	Complete. Pre-filters added. The respirators provide protection superior to what the most stringent requirement in the proposed OSHA standard.
10	Enhance current Respiratory Protection Program.	Identify hazardous chemicals requiring respiratory protection. Identify type of respirator and cartridge for each chemical. Add specific list of chemical and respirator needed into the existing program.	11-Jun-09	Complete.
11	Respiratory protection during formulation process.	Change procedure to wear respirator during full weighing cycle. Obtain chronological test data for exposures after weighing.	23-Jun-09 31-Jul-09	Complete. Implemented procedural change for respirator use. IH sample results to be evaluated. A second survey is planned in September to confirm the first set of results.
12	Evaluate spill response procedures.	Review existing procedures and revise to include handling of spills by emergency response with appropriate PPE (Tyvek suits, butyl gloves) and disposal of contaminated materials.	16-Jun-09	Completed procedure review. New standard communicated to first responder personnel. The procedure will be revised and communicated to all personnel by mid-September.
13	Establish cleaning procedures to minimize airborne diacetyl.	Initiate use of cold water for cleaning.	12-Jun-09	Complete.
14	Health hazard training on diacetyl for employees. Health warnings on MSDS and labels.	Develop training materials, incorporate into existing Hazcom and Respiratory Protection programs. Continue to update MSDS. Train employees annually.	18-Jun-09	Complete. MSDS's health hazards are updated/entered as they are reviewed/developed.

Table 10. (continued)

Item No.	Action Item	Proposed Action	Estimated Completion Date	Status
15	Use of engineering control ventilation by production employees.	Develop training material, train all personnel, and document training.	31-Jul-09	Complete. Training completed for manufacturing. The total diacetyl handling procedure (which includes this particular item) will be reviewed with both manufacturing and R&D per action item 28.
16	Use OSHA methods 1012 & 1013 for IH testing.	Have IH consultant use OSHA methods.	09-Mar-09	Complete.
17	Substitutes for diacetyl.	Define possible means of removing diacetyl and substitutes for future formulations.	TBD	Policy implemented to avoid diacetyl in new formulations wherever possible.
18	Hazcom training specific to diacetyl.	Develop training module.	18-Jun-09	Complete.
19	Enhance recordkeeping - Medical form consistent with proposed OSHA standard.	Develop form containing employee work history, spirometry testing results, employee communications, etc.	22-Jun-09	Complete.
20	Make the December 2003 NIOSH Alert available to all employees.	Determine best means of accomplishing or if past practices have met the equivalency of doing so.	24-Jun-09	Complete. Past practice was probably sufficient but now enhanced.
21	Evaluate addition order of diacetyl containing batches.	Determine if diacetyl can be the last component added to a batch to minimize total potential exposure period.	07-Jul-09	Complete.
22	Conduct communication session on diacetyl and IH issues with all employees.	Communicate proposed new OSHA standard and steps taken by company to be in full compliance.	20-Jul-09	Complete.
23	Evaluate need for refrigerated storage with closed dispensing system.	Determine vapor pressure at various storage temperatures. Analyze likely effect of storage temperature change on personnel exposures.	07-Jul-09	Complete. Procedure implemented to refrigerate diacetyl until used.
24	Review monitoring data collected during June and July.	Conduct meeting to analyze data to date and formulate an action plan to address findings.	05-Aug-09	Complete. No issues in packaging, SOD, and R&D relative to most conservative proposed OSHA permissible exposure limit of 50 ppb. Closed pumping system in X-oil room successful in reducing exposure levels to well below 50 ppb. Spray Dry, Reactions, and Liquid Compounding areas will be studied further.
25	Repeat study to confirm positive impact of the closed pumping system in the X-oil room.	Conduct a second round of testing with the new pump system to see whether positive results from first test can be duplicated.	15-Sep-09	
26	Monitor Spray Dry, Reactions, and Liquid Compounding areas.	Schedule IH survey under controlled processing conditions to define sources of exposure and evaluate options for containment.	21-Sep-09	The study will include investigation of the transfer process, the operating conditions (temperature, pressure), and any other relevant factors that may contribute to higher concentrations. This evaluation will pinpoint the sources and define the means of mitigation/elimination.
27	Summarize data to date and action plan going forward and communicate to site employees.	Develop chart with a summary of current results by area. The chart will reflect averages and range of results.	28-Aug-09	
28	Complete training for all site personnel on handling procedures, which fully incorporate specifics in the proposed OSHA standard.	Finalize procedures and schedule training for all site personnel.	30-Sep-09	

Regarding our interim report recommendation to take precautions similar to those for diacetyl if diacetyl substitutes are used, the company implemented a policy to avoid diacetyl and substitutes in new product formulations whenever possible (Table 10). Additionally, they were going to determine, when diacetyl is used, if it could be added as the last component of the batch to minimize potential for exposure to diacetyl.

The company initiated cold water cleaning and cold storage of diacetyl per our recommendations. Table 10 also indicates that they successfully developed a closed dispensing system in the X-Oil room with reduction in diacetyl exposure levels. Further study was planned for installation in other areas such as spray dry and liquid compounding.

Respiratory protection

Fifty-three employees with information from 2007 and/or 2008 had been medically cleared to wear respirators.

Although the initial respiratory protection program documentation received prior to our visit covered respirator maintenance, selection, inspection, and use in the workplace, it did not include clear guidelines on when to wear respirators. Our interim report included a recommendation that a list of chemicals and their corresponding respirator selection and filter/cartridge selection criteria be incorporated into the written respiratory protection program so that employees understand exactly when and for what chemicals respiratory protection is required. The August 2009 respiratory protection program documentation included, in its table of respiratory equipment used at the facility, the addition of full-face respirators with organic vapor and particulate filter cartridges for use when dispensing diacetyl. However, the table included descriptions of other respirators without information on the associated hazardous chemicals or job titles and tasks for which that respirator should be worn.

During our site visit, we noticed that production batch tickets indicated the need for respiratory protection for some chemicals during the first use of the chemical in the process, but there was no indication of the need for respiratory protection for those same chemicals on subsequent batch tickets. We also observed that only the employee working directly with a chemical wore respiratory protection while an employee in close proximity did not. The action items prepared by the company in 2009 (Table 10) indicated that the recommendation in our interim report to require respiratory protection in downstream batches was incorporated into the full weighing cycle, and air sampling results would be evaluated to determine the downstream need after weighing. An action item in response to our recommendation to require respiratory protection for employees in close proximity to exposed employees was not included.

In response to our interim report recommendation that employees wear respirators and eye and skin protection when cleaning spills or washing empty containers of flavoring chemicals, an action item in Table 10 indicated that the company would prepare a revised procedure to include handling of spills by emergency response personnel with appropriate personal protective equipment.

Hazard communication

The two MSDSs we reviewed during our site visit for diacetyl-containing products referred to the "December 2003 NIOSH Report" (presumably the December 2003 NIOSH Alert, "Preventing Lung Disease in Employees Who Use or Make Flavorings") on the occurrence of severe lung disease in employees who make or use flavorings. In our interim report, we recommended that the company make the NIOSH Alert available to their medical provider and their own employees. The company's action items in Table 10 indicate that although they considered their past practice as sufficient, they enhanced it. Regarding our other recommendations for communication of diacetyl and diacetyl substitute health hazard information to its employees, the company's action items indicate they developed a diacetyl training module for presentation in annual training sessions. Information in the training sessions was to include health hazards, air sampling results, company action items, proper use of LEV hoods and respirators, and flavoring handling procedures.

DISCUSSION

The additional spirometry screening results provided by the company after our June 2009 interim letter were consistent with our previous findings: Its employees had nearly four times the prevalence of spirometric restriction than the general United States population, after adjusting for contributing factors such as overweight and obesity. Eight of the 25 employees with spirometric restriction and serial spirometry measurements had abnormal declines of spirometry measured over time, consistent with progressive loss during employment. The statistical associations that we have documented between abnormal declines in lung function and jobs with high potential for flavorings exposures suggest employment exposures may be causing deterioration in lung health. The finding that 37% of employees had either abnormal spirometry or abnormal declines in spirometry or both is concerning. Putting in place a program that identifies employees who have abnormal rates of decline in spirometry on serial testing but still have normal FEV_1 and FVC values may offer the opportunity to intervene early and preserve normal lung function.

The analyses presented here suggest that these abnormal rates of lung function decline are related to workplace exposures. The evidence in favor of work-relatedness is three-fold: First, employees with higher potential for flavorings exposure in their work areas had 2.8 times greater annualized decline in FEV_1 than employees in jobs with lower potential for exposure, and the average yearly decline was about 4 times greater than is normal in the general population (124 versus 30 ml/year). Second, employees with current higher potential for flavorings exposure had 7 times the risk of abnormal decline in FEV_1 compared to employees with lower potential for exposure. Because employees often relocate to other jobs if they have or suspect health effects related to their work ("healthy worker effect"), we evaluated whether employees who had ever worked in areas with higher potential for flavorings exposure had higher risk compared to employees who had never worked in areas with higher potential for exposure and found even higher risk than was associated with current employment in potential high exposure jobs. Finally, within the higher potential for flavorings exposure work areas, we could demonstrate that a single job group, those ever working in liquid compounding, had statistically increased annual FEV_1 decline in comparison to employees who never worked in areas with higher potential flavorings exposures. With these three types of evidence for excessive deterioration in pulmonary function associated with employment in areas with high potential for flavorings exposure, the company needs to aggressively intervene to assure that its employees are protected from potentially harmful exposures.

We do not think that the absence of a statistical association between restrictive abnormality and work areas with higher potential for flavorings exposure is evidence against a work-related excess of restriction. The employees referred for spirometric testing were all thought to have potential for flavorings exposure, which is documented in the diacetyl measurements available from the company's 2009 sampling. Thus, the 3.8-fold excess of restriction in the employee population undergoing surveillance compared to the general population was broadly distributed between areas that we thought had higher potential for flavorings exposure and areas that had lower potential for flavorings exposure. The maximum diacetyl exposures documented in some of the employees working in lower potential for exposure areas were high enough to have caused lung disease in microwave popcorn plant employees [Kanwal et al. 2006]. We do not know that diacetyl is the cause of the lung disease in this company's flavoring employees. Cases of flavoring-related lung disease in microwave popcorn employees suggests that a susceptible subpopulation exists that develops disease within months and at relatively low exposures compared to mixers [Akpinar-Elci et al. 2004; Kreiss et al. 2002].

Understandably, both the company and medical contractor were concerned by the potential respiratory hazard of diacetyl. These concerns were evident in the efforts of the company to decrease diacetyl exposure through respiratory protection, changes in work practices, substitution of diacetyl by other chemicals, and education of employees about specifics that had been proposed for inclusion in a possible Occupational Safety and Health Administration standard for diacetyl (Table 10).

However, flavoring companies have many chemical exposures other than diacetyl. Thus, even though restrictive spirometric abnormalities are not normally thought to be a result of diacetyl exposure, our evidence of increased burden of restriction in the work force, accelerated rate of FEV_1 decline, and statistical associations between this decline and work history should motivate additional efforts to evaluate potential causes and control potentially causative exposures.

The first step should be to determine the nature of the restrictive spirometric abnormalities seen in nearly one-third of employees with usable spirometry. As indicated above, restriction may reflect obesity, but we adjusted for body mass index in both comparisons with the U.S. population and in models of excess risk by job indices of exposure. We also adjusted for change in weight over the spirometry intervals in looking at the declines in FEV_1, which paralleled the declines in FVC, as would be expected in evolving restrictive abnormalities. Another cause of spirometric restriction is neuromuscular weakness, but this seems an unlikely cause in a production employee population. Poor quality spirometry with insufficient inhalation before forced expiration or insufficient exhalation time and effort can result in apparent restrictive abnormalities, but we limited our analyses to spirometry with adequate repeatability within test sessions. Despite our care in evaluating the data, it is certainly possible that some individual employees may have had these non-pulmonary causes of a restrictive spirometric pattern. However, our analysis suggests that most of the restrictive abnormalities documented in the work force are not due to obesity or artifacts related to poor test quality.

Instead, we are concerned that these changes in spirometry may reflect underlying scarring or inflammatory (interstitial) occupational lung disease in a substantial fraction of company employees with abnormal spirometry. Additional diagnostic tests other than spirometry are needed to establish the proportion of employees with restrictive spirometry that have low lung volumes or other evidence of interstitial lung disease. The predictive value of a restrictive pattern of spirometry for low lung volumes in a population of patients referred to a hospital pulmonary function laboratory was 58% [Aaron et al. 1999]. The prevalence rate of true restriction documented by lung volume testing might be higher in the company's employees, given their common exposures that might be a cause of restrictive lung disease. Still, without medical testing in addition to spirometry, we cannot be sure whether spirometric restriction reflects lung disease. It should be noted that in a case series of patients with documented restrictive lung diseases, the combination of restrictive spirometry and low total lung capacity were quite insensitive [Boros et al. 2004]. Thus, if true restrictive lung disease is shown to exist in some employees with restrictive spirometry, all employees may need to have other diagnostic tests performed to assess for interstitial lung disease.

All employees with abnormal current spirometry (including restrictive, obstructive, and mixed abnormalities) or excessive declines in FEV_1 need evaluation with further medical tests by an appropriate specialist with expertise in occupational and pulmonary medicine who is knowledgeable about this report and its findings. Steps for follow up evaluation of those with restrictive spirometric abnormalities might include confirming restriction by measuring lung volumes; evaluating gas transport by measuring carbon monoxide diffusing capacity; testing for exercise-induced oxygen desaturation; and evaluation with sensitive imaging studies such as high resolution computerized tomography scanning. For those with obstructive abnormalities, steps for follow up evaluation might include evaluating for spirometric bronchodilator response, measuring lung volumes to assess for air trapping, ruling out emphysematous or interstitial changes by measuring carbon monoxide diffusing capacity, and evaluation of paired inspiratory and expiratory high resolution computerized tomography scans for evidence of air trapping. Evaluating the 10 employees with moderate to very severe spirometric abnormalities first may be particularly informative about potential disease processes and could guide subsequent diagnostic evaluation of those with mild abnormalities. Specialist attention might also be useful in evaluating for excessive spirometric decline on an ongoing basis, using the information to intervene early to reduce potential workplace exposures while employees still have relatively normal lung function.

Restrictive abnormalities have previously been documented among flavoring-exposed employees in other work settings. Although diacetyl and flavoring exposures are well known to have caused crippling lung disease due to fixed obstruction and bronchiolitis obliterans in the microwave popcorn and flavoring manufacturing industries, the full spectrum of lung diseases related to flavoring exposures remains unclear [Kreiss 2007a]. A case of restrictive lung disease without a nonoccupational explanation has been reported among former employees in the index microwave popcorn plant [Akpinar-Elci et al. 2004]. Cases of restriction were present early in the investigation [Kreiss et al. 2002] and evolved during follow-up [NIOSH 2006]. Restriction has also been noted in other microwave popcorn plants [NIOSH 2003]. In flavoring manufacturing employees in California, there were more employees with restrictive than with obstructive spirometric abnormalities [Kim et al. 2010]. One case report documents restrictive spirometry in a food production plant worker who used flavorings. He was found to have bronchiolitis obliterans with organizing pneumonia [Alleman and Darcy 2002]. In another report, 4 of 22 food production plant workers had spirometric restriction. None of the 22 had obstruction [Day et al. 2011]. Thus, while the significance of restrictive lung disease among flavorings-exposed workers remains uncertain, current medical literature suggests that it may be within the spectrum of health effects related to flavorings exposure.

The current report documents an excess of employees with restrictive spirometry and an association between longitudinal loss of lung function and employment in certain job categories. The finding that abnormal loss of lung function is not uniformly distributed among company employees and is concentrated among employees with higher potential for flavoring exposures is consistent with a work-related cause. To understand what is causing these abnormalities and how to address them, the company's medical contractor needs access to employees' further diagnostic tests. Company referral of workers needing in-depth evaluations to a small group of expert medical consultants might facilitate rapid recognition of disease patterns so that the spectrum of flavoring-related disease can be established. Similarly, physicians conducting ongoing medical surveillance should have access to job, area, and task information so that they can recognize epidemiologic patterns of abnormalities and their distribution in the employee population, facilitating recognition of work-related adverse health effects and ongoing targeting of prevention efforts.

Because symptoms of respiratory disease may not be reported by employees, medical surveillance including spirometry is essential to protecting employees' health. The company should work with its medical provider to establish a formal medical monitoring and surveillance program. The California Department of Public Health, with assistance from NIOSH, developed guidelines for medical surveillance for flavoring-related lung disease among flavoring manufacturing employees [California 2007]. The guidelines recommend that once an employee is identified as having a flavoring-related lung disease, employees whose jobs pose similar or greater risk should undergo spirometry testing every 3 months. In this facility, there is both excess spirometric restriction compared to the general population and evidence of work-related excessive decline in FEV_1. Although the nature of these abnormalities is unclear, we recommend testing at 3-month intervals until the nature of the excessive FEV_1 declines among production employees is understood and abnormal declines stabilize following lowered exposures. More frequent testing provides an opportunity for the medical provider to improve spirometry quality, which is critical for early ascertainment of excessive declines. In World Trade Center responder medical surveillance, the criterion for adequate technician performance is that 80% of employees achieve A or B quality spirometry [Enright et al. 2010]. In fact, even 90% of ill patients can achieve A or B quality spirometry with adequate coaching [Enright et al. 2004]. In comparison, the medical contractor providing spirometry to this company achieved 62% A or B quality on company employees. Suboptimal quality (including C, D, and F quality) spirometry should be repeated within a month. The company might consider withholding payment for spirometry testing in which quality criteria are not met.

There are several limitations in our evaluation of this plant. First, 19% of the spirometry records provided by the company's medical provider were of D or F quality, and an additional 18 % had C quality, indicating marginal repeatability of measurements within a test session. High quality spirometry testing improves the ability to detect relationships between exposures and employees' lung function, particularly in evaluating declines over time. Our evaluation of serial spirometry records may have underestimated abnormal declines because we excluded poor quality spirometry, and only 70 employees had serial tests with A, B, or C quality. The work history information provided by the company was less detailed than we would have collected from direct employee interviews to identify high-risk tasks associated with job titles. Data analysis was based on limited observations of the various processes performed at this facility, and few exposure measurements were available to support our classification of some areas as having higher potential for flavoring exposures than the remainder of jobs and areas. These limitations may have resulted in misclassification of exposures and health outcomes, either of which would lower our ability to detect possible work related associations. For example, we did not include laboratory, research and development and quality control, and packaging employees in the group with higher potential for exposure, although this classification would be appropriate in some other plants that we have visited.

Unavailability of quantitative exposure characterization for employees in various work areas over time prevented us from doing more sophisticated statistical analyses concerning the relationship between cumulative or average exposure estimates from a job-exposure matrix linked to work history and lung function abnormalities. Representative exposure assessments in flavorings plants are difficult because of the wide diversity in batch operations and recipes. On our walk through of the plant, the NIOSH industrial hygienist and engineer collected only four air samples on the second shift for an hour or less. These few samples were not intended to be representative of workplace exposures overall. NIOSH did not have relative humidity, temperature, and days to extraction with which to correct company air sampling data collected between March 2004 and July 2007 using NIOSH Method 2557, which is known to be affected by absolute humidity and time to extraction of sampling media. The company air sampling data provided to NIOSH following our site visit was collected using OSHA sampling methods that require no adjustment. Although we could not construct a job-exposure matrix over time with the available company data, the more recent company measurements provided some evidence that the areas that we considered to have higher potential for flavoring exposures had higher diacetyl measurements. No measurements were available for extract and distillation, which had no current employee and only one past employee.

A final limitation is the small numbers of employees in many production categories. Small numbers limit statistical power to determine differences among subgroups. We were able to demonstrate that employees who ever worked in liquid compounding had significantly greater declines in FEV_1 compared to employees who had never worked in areas with high potential for exposures to flavorings. This statistical finding does not imply that employees in other areas within the group of higher potential exposure areas had no risk, but whatever risk they might have could not be detected with the numbers of employees. We were not able to demonstrate that restrictive abnormalities were associated with working in an area with higher potential for exposure. Whether this was the result of inadequate power to detect a difference, misclassification of exposure or health response, or no association cannot be determined. However, the constellation of excessive restrictive spirometry in the whole population, work-related excessive FEV_1 decline, and uncertainty about the levels of safe exposures to an unknown causal agent(s) present in this workplace present cause for concern and justify measures to assure that potential respiratory health problems are recognized, characterized, and prevented.

CONCLUSIONS

The findings from our spirometry record review indicate that the flavorings manufacturing facility employees who underwent spirometry testing at the contracted clinic had 3.8 times greater prevalence of spirometric restriction than the U.S. population after adjusting for age, gender, race, smoking, and body mass index. About one-third of employees had spirometric abnormalities, most of them restrictive in nature. Furthermore, even using the conservative criteria recommended by ACOEM, 17% of the employees with adequate longitudinal spirometry data had abnormal declines in FEV_1 over time. Statistical modeling indicated that abnormal decline in FEV_1 and that annualized average decreases in FEV_1 and FVC were associated with working in areas with higher potential for exposure to flavoring chemicals. Employees who had ever done liquid processing had greater average annualized falls in spirometric measurements than employees who had never worked in an area with higher potential for flavoring exposure. These results suggest that the flavorings company employees are experiencing respiratory health effects related to ongoing exposures in the workplace. Further medical testing of those with abnormalities in spirometry is warranted to define any lung diseases resulting in restrictive spirometric abnormality in this workplace. Frequent follow-up of those with excessive FEV_1 decline may assist in documenting that workplace interventions to lower flavoring exposure are effective in preventing work-associated declines in lung function.

RECOMMENDATIONS

Based on observations and findings from our initial site visit and subsequent documentation we received, we encourage the company to continue to use the recommendations provided in our interim report. Following are additional recommendations; some may appear to repeat those previously provided because we lack information on the status of action items, or to emphasize the importance of continuing consideration:

Substitution and engineering controls

1. Until inhalation toxicity information is available on diacetyl substitutes such as acetoin, 2,3-pentanedione, 2,3-hexanedione, 2,3-heptanedione, starter distillate (which contains diacetyl), and diacetyl trimer (which decomposes to diacetyl), the same precautions needed to prevent diacetyl exposure need to be taken for these substitutes.

2. The local exhaust ventilation hoods should be evaluated periodically to assess their performance and to identify any design or operational deficiencies.

3. Continue to avoid use of floor fans in the vicinity of hooded processes, as the floor fans could disturb the airflow and dramatically reduce the effectiveness of local exhaust hoods, particularly the moveable exhaust hoods.

4. Continue to keep production areas where flavors are compounded under lower room air pressure than adjacent areas. This reduces the escape of flavoring chemicals and potential exposure to other areas.

Respiratory protection

5. A list of chemicals and their corresponding respirator and filter/cartridge selection criteria should be incorporated into the written respiratory protection program. Specific guidance is necessary for employees to understand exactly what chemicals and tasks pose exposure hazards, which employees are at risk, and what respirator will provide adequate protection.

6. Batch tickets should reflect the need to wear appropriate respiratory protection throughout the flavor formulation process, regardless of the process step. Although use of respiratory protection was extended to weighing tasks, as well as during the first use of the chemical, downstream exposures to intermediate mixtures of chemicals during subsequent batch tickets may also require respiratory protection.

7. Because chemicals such as diacetyl are volatile and can easily migrate from one location to other nearby locations, nearby employees should employ proper respirators.

8. Continue to have employees wear personal protection equipment including: (1) respirators that provide protection against both organic vapors and particulates and (2) eye and skin protection when cleaning up spills or washing empty containers of flavoring chemicals or ingredients.

Hazard communication / employee education

9. Because the plant manufactures food flavorings, the company should make copies of the December 2003

"NIOSH Alert: Preventing lung disease in employees who use or make flavorings" available to their medical provider and to their own employees.

10. The company should continue updating its MSDSs with information on diacetyl health hazards and means of protection, and providing respiratory protection guidelines on production batch labels. We also encourage the company to keep their training module up to date on the health hazards of and protection from flavoring chemicals (including diacetyl). These should comply with OSHA Hazard Communication guidance for diacetyl and other flavoring ingredients (http://www.osha.gov/dsg/guidance/diacetyl-guidance.html). If diacetyl substitutes are introduced, we suggest that the MSDSs, training, respiratory protection, and work practices incorporate similar protective measures because the respiratory toxicity of diacetyl substitutes remains unclear.

11. Continue to ensure that employees are trained on how to use the local exhaust ventilation hoods properly; provide guidance on proper usage and good work practices.

12. Continue to keep containers of flavoring chemicals and/or ingredients sealed when not in use, and use cold water washes and cold storage of chemicals when feasible.

Medical screening and surveillance

13. The company should work together with its medical provider to establish a formal medical monitoring and surveillance program. This program should include ascertainment of symptoms and spirometry testing of lung function for all employees with potentially hazardous exposure to flavorings or flavoring ingredients prior to job placement and then every 3 months. Since high quality spirometry is critical to determining excessive declines in FEV_1, the company might consider incentives to its contractor to achieve the highest quality spirometry possible. When the company has evidence that excessive declines in lung function in the workforce have resolved with good quality serial spirometry, the interval for assessment of symptoms and spirometry testing of exposed employees can be increased to every 6 months. The monitoring and surveillance program should identify cases of lung function abnormalities among flavorings-exposed employees, establish baseline measurements for new employees, and

track changes in lung function over time to detect any rapid or excessive decline in lung function. NIOSH SPIROLA software is available without cost to assist in tracking abnormal declines in spirometry. Detecting abnormal declines in lung function is essential to prevent employees from suffering harm which may be irreversible. Those with abnormalities in spirometry or excessive interval declines in FEV_1 should be evaluated further for diagnosis and appropriate management, considered for work restriction from further flavoring exposure, and followed at 3 month intervals until stable.

The company's contract with its medical provider should provide for aggregate epidemiologic analysis of the medical results, including analysis of medical results by department or job. Aggregate analysis can identify hazards associated with flavoring manufacture and may assist the company with data-driven priorities for prevention through exposure control. Medical results considered in aggregate analyses should include both the results of the medical monitoring and surveillance program; and the results of any in-depth medical evaluations resulting from abnormal findings identified by the monitoring and surveillance program. Company referral of employees needing in-depth evaluations to a small group of expert medical consultants might facilitate rapid recognition and reporting of disease patterns suggesting emerging workforce health problems.

Exposure assessment

14. For air sampling, continue to use OSHA Methods 1012 and 1013 to measure diacetyl in the air (http://www.osha.gov/dts/sltc/methods/validated/1012/1012.html and http://www.osha.gov/dts/sltc/methods/validated/1013/1013.html). Routine measurements should be made to ensure continued engineering control effectiveness in preventing diacetyl exposures. Additional measurements should be obtained following changes in processes or controls that could affect exposures to diacetyl. In the absence of regulated permissible exposure limits, flavoring exposures should be as low as possible, since health-protective exposures may be lower than analytic limits of detection.

REFERENCES

Aaron SD, Dales RE, Cardinal [1999]. How accurate is spirometry at predicting restrictive pulmonary impairment? Chest 115:869-873.

Akpinar-Elci M, Travis WD, Lynch DA, Kreiss K [2004]. Bronchiolitis obliterans syndrome in popcorn production plant workers. Eur Respir J 24(2):298-302. http://www.ncbi.nlm.nih.gov/pubmed/15332401

Alleman T, and Darcey D [2002]. Case report: Bronchiolitis obliterans organizing pneumonia in a spice process technician. J Occup Environ Med 44(3):215-216.

Boros PW, Franczuk M, Wesolowski S [2004].Value of spirometry in detecting volume restriction in interstitial lung disease patients. Respir 71:374-379.

California Department of Public Health [2007]. Medical surveillance for flavorings-related lung disease among flavoring manufacturing workers in California. Occupational Health Branch, California Department of Public Health. [http://www.cdph.ca.gov/programs/ohb/Documents/flavor-guidelines. pdf]. Date accessed: March 2011.

Cox-Ganser J, Ganser G, Saito R, Hobbs G, Boylstein R, Hendricks W, Simmons M, Eide M, Kullman G, Piacitelli C [2011]. Correcting diacetyl concentrations from air samples collected with NIOSH Method 2557. J Occup Environ Hyg 8(2):59-70.

Day G, Lebouf R, Grote A, Pendergrass S, Cummings K, Kreiss K, Kullman G [2011]. Identification and measurement of diacetyl substitutes in dry bakery mix production. J Occup Environ Hyg 8:93-103.

Enright PL, Beck KC, Sherrill DL [2004]. Repeatability of spirometry in 18,000 adult patients. Am J Respir Crit Care Med 169:235-238.

Enright PL, Skloot GS, Cox-Ganser JM, Udasin IG, Herbert R [2010]. Quality of spirometry performed by 13,599 participants in the World Trade Center worker and volunteer medical screening program. Respir Care 55(3):303-309.

Flavor and Extract Manufacturers Association [2004]. Respiratory Health and Safety in the Flavor Manufacturing Workplace. The Flavor and Extract Manufacturers Association of the United States, Washington, D.C.

Hankinson J, Odencrantz J, Fedan K [1999]. Spirometric reference values from a sample of the general U.S. population. Am J Respir Crit Care Med 159:179-187.

Hnizdo E, Yan T, Hakobyan A, Enright P, Beeckman-Wagner LA, Hankinson J, Fleming J, Lee Petsonk E [2010]. Spirometry Longitudinal Data Analysis Software (SPIROLA) for analysis of spirometry data in workplace prevention or COPD treatment. Open Med Inform J 4:94-102.

Hubbs AF, Goldsmith WT, Kashon ML, Frazer D, Mercer RR, Battelli LA, Kullman GJ, Schwegler-Berry D, Friend S, Castranova V [2008]. Respiratory toxicologic pathology of inhaled diacetyl in sprague-dawley rats. Toxicol Pathol 36(2):330-44.

Kanwal R, Kullman G, Piacitelli C, Boylstein R, Sahakian N, Martin S, Fedan K, Kreiss K [2006]. Evaluation of flavorings-related lung disease risk at six microwave popcorn plants. J Occup Environ Med 48(2):149-157.

Kim T, Materna B, Prudhomme J, Fedan K, Enright P, Sahakian N, Windham G, Kreiss K [2010]. Industry-wide medical surveillance of California flavor manufacturing workers: cross-sectional results. Am J Ind Med 53:857-865.

Kreiss K [2007a]. Flavoring-related bronchiolitis obliterans. Curr Opin Allergy Clin Immunol 7:162-167.

Kreiss K [2007b]. Occupational bronchiolitis obliterans masquerading as COPD. Am J Respir Crit Care Med 176:427-429.

Kreiss K, Gomaa A, Kullman G, Fedan K, Simoes EJ, Enright PL [2002]. Clinical bronchiolitis obliterans in workers at a microwave popcorn plant. N Engl J Med 347(5):330-338.

Kullman G, Boylstein R, Jones W, Piacitelli C, Pendergrass S, Kreiss K [2005]. Characterization of respiratory exposures at a microwave popcorn plant with cases of bronchiolitis obliterans. J Occup Environ Hyg 2:169-178.

National Center for Health Statistics [1996]. Third National Health and Nutrition Examination Survey, 1988-1994, National Health and Nutrition Examination Survey III laboratory data file. Public use data file documentation number 76200. Hyattsville, MD: Centers for Disease Control and Prevention, 1996 (CD-ROM).

NIOSH [2003]. Hazard evaluation and technical assistance report: Agrilink Foods Popcorn Plant, Ridgway, IL. By Sahakian N, Choe K, Boylstein R, Schleiff P. U.S. Department of Health and Human Services, Centers for Disease Control and Prevention, National Institute for Occupational Safety and Health, NIOSH HETA Report No. 2002-0408-2915.

NIOSH [2004]. NIOSH alert: preventing lung disease in workers who use or make flavorings. By Kanwal R, Kullman K, Kreiss K, Castellan R, Burkhart J, Hilsbos K, Akpinar-Elci M, Piacitelli C, Boylstein R. U.S. Department of Health and Human Services, Centers for Disease Control and Prevention, National Institute for Occupational Safety and Health, DHHS (NIOSH) Publication Number 2004-110.

NIOSH [2006]. Hazard evaluation and technical assistance report: Gilster-Mary Lee Corporation, Jasper, MO. By Kanwal R, Kullman G, Fedan K, Kreiss K. U.S. Department of Health and Human Services, Centers for Disease Control and Prevention, National Institute for Occupational Safety and Health.

NIOSH HETA Report No. 2000-0401-2991.

NIOSH [2008]. NIOSH manual of analytical methods (NMAM®). 4th ed. Schlecht PC, O'Connor PF, eds. Cincinnati, OH: U.S. Department of Health and Human Services, Centers for Disease Control and Prevention, National Institute for Occupational safety and Health, DHHS (NIOSH) Publication 94–113 (August 1994); 1st Supplement Publication 96–135, 2nd Supplement Publication 98–119; 3rd Supplement 2003–154. [http://www.cdc.gov/niosh/docs/2003-154/].

Pellegrino R, Viegi G, Brusasco V, Crapo RO, Burgos F, Casaburi R, Coates A, van der Grinten CP, Gustafsson P, Hankinson J, Jensen R, Johnson DC, MacIntyre N, McKay R, Miller MR, Navajas D, Pedersen OF, Wanger J [2005]. Interpretative strategies for lung function tests. Eur Respir J 26:948–968.

Sherrill DL, Lebowitz MD, Knudson RJ, Burrows B [1992]. Continuous longitudinal regression equations for pulmonary function measures. Eur Respir J 5:452-462.

Wang ML, Petsonk EL [2004]. Repeated measures of FEV_1 over six to twelve months: What change is abnormal? J Occup Environ Med 46:591-595.

Wang ML, Avashia BH, Petsonk EL [2006]. Interpreting periodic lung function tests in individuals. Chest 130:493-499.

ACKNOWLEDGEMENTS AND AVAILABILITY OF REPORT

The Respiratory Disease Hazard Evaluation and Technical Assistance Program (RDHETAP) of NIOSH conducts field investigations of possible health hazards in the workplace. These investigations are conducted under the authority of Section 20(a)(6) of the Occupational Safety and Health (OSH) Act of 1970, 29 U.S.C. 669(a)(6), or Section 501(a)(11) of the Federal Mine Safety and Health Act of 1977, 30 U.S.C. 951(a)(11), which authorizes the Secretary of Health and Human Services, following a written request from any employers or authorized representative of employees, to determine whether any substance normally found in the place of employment has potentially toxic effects in such concentrations as used or found.

RDHETAP also provides, upon request, technical and consultative assistance to federal, state, and local agencies; labor; industry; and other groups or individuals to control occupational health hazards and to prevent related trauma and disease.

Mention of any company or product does not constitute endorsement by NIOSH. In addition, citations to websites external to NIOSH do not constitute NIOSH endorsement of the sponsoring organizations or their programs or products. Furthermore, NIOSH is not responsible for the content of these websites. All Web addresses referenced in this document were accessible as of the publication date.

This report was prepared by Kay Kreiss, Jean Cox-Ganser, and Chris Piacitelli of RDHETAP, Division of Respiratory Disease Studies. Field site visit was conducted by Yulia Iossifova, Nancy Sahakian, James Couch, and Kevin H. Dunn. Data management and programming was provided by Brian Tift, Kathy Fedan, Nicole Edwards, and Carrie Thomas. Pulmonary function interpretation was aided by Paul Enright, M D. Desktop publishing was performed by Tia McClelland.

Copies of this report have been sent to management representatives at the facility, HHE requestor (local branch of the International Brotherhood of Teamsters), the Indiana State Department of Health, and the OSHA Region 5 Office. This report is not copyrighted and may be freely reproduced. The report may be viewed and printed from the following internet address: http://www.cdc.gov/niosh/hhe. Copies may be purchased from the National Technical Information Service (NTIS) at 5825 Port Royal Road, Springfield, Virginia 22161.

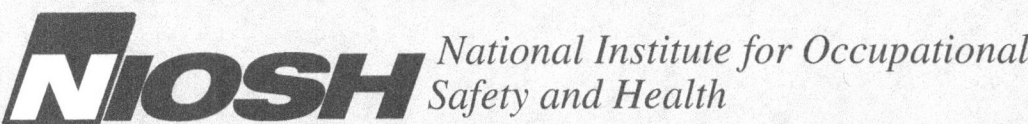

National Institute for Occupational Safety and Health

Delivering on the Nation's promise: Safety and health at work for all people through research and prevention.

To receive NIOSH documents or information about occupational safety and health topics contact NIOSH at:

1-800-35-NIOSH (1-800-356-4674)

Fax: 1-513-533-8573

E-mail: pubstaft@cdc.gov
or visit the NIOSH web site at:
http://www.cdc.gov/niosh/hhe

SAFER • HEALTHIER • PEOPLE™

www.ingramcontent.com/pod-product-compliance
Lightning Source LLC
Chambersburg PA
CBHW080915290526
45795CB00007BA/2526